KAREEMA BAKSH

The Transformative Touch of Cancer on My Existence

A Journey of Healing and Restoring the Mind, Body, and Spirit

Dedication

To my daughter Shivanna and granddaughter Zarah, who have inspired significant shifts in my lifestyle. Zarah, may you one day understand the struggles I faced and learn from my experiences.

To my four supportive sisters, whose love and presence I deeply cherish.

To my parents, especially my father, for providing a good life and encouraging me to pursue excellence and education.

To my friends and healthcare providers for your unwavering support.

With love and light.

"The wound is the place where the Light enters you."
– Rumi

"Out of difficulties grow miracles."
– Jean de La Bruyère

"In the midst of winter, I found there was, within me, an invincible summer."
– Albert Camus

"Per Ardua Ad Astra" (Through difficulties to Success)
– Royal Air Force Motto

Contents

I

Introduction

Life was moving along as usual, a blend of daily routines, personal goals, and the occasional surprise that kept things interesting. Yet, nothing could have prepared me for the moment that would redefine everything I knew about existence
when my world was turned upside down with three simple words: "You have Cancer"
This is my story, a testament to the transformational power of facing life's greatest challenges head-on, and emerging not just as a survivor, but as a warrior of light and love!

1

The Purpose of Cancer

Cancer. The mere mention of the word can send shivers down the spine, evoking images of hospital rooms, endless treatments, and uncertain futures. For many, cancer is synonymous with fear, suffering, and loss. But what if we dared to look beyond the pain and fear? What if we asked ourselves a deeper question: What is the purpose of cancer?

In embarking on this journey, I was forced to confront this question head-on. Initially, my diagnosis felt like a cruel twist of fate, an uninvited guest that barged into my life and turned everything upside down. I felt lost, overwhelmed, and frightened. However, as I navigated the labyrinth of medical appointments, treatments, and the roller coaster of emotions that accompanied them, a shift began to occur within me. I started to see cancer not just as an adversary, but as a profound teacher! It came into my life to teach me a lesson and force me onto a new path ...

The purpose of cancer, as I have come to understand, is multifaceted. It is a call to pause, reflect, and reassess our lives. It forces us to confront our vulnerabilities and our strengths, to re-evaluate our priorities, and to seek out the deeper meaning to our existence. In many ways, cancer strips away the superficial layers of our lives, revealing the raw, unvarnished truth of who we are and what truly matters.

Firstly, cancer serves as a powerful reminder of our mortality. It is a stark acknowledgment that life is finite, and that time is a precious, non-renewable resource. This realization can be both terrifying and liberating. It compels us to live more fully in the present moment, to cherish our relationships, and to pursue our passions with renewed vigor. When faced with the fragility of life, we are prompted to let go of trivial concerns and to focus on what brings us genuine joy and fulfillment.

For many, including myself, this confrontation with mortality ignites a spiritual awakening. It invites us to explore the deeper, often unspoken questions about our existence: Why are we here? What is our purpose? How can we find peace and meaning in the face of SUFFERING ?

The Buddha teaches that life is full of suffering and that there is a cause for this suffering !

These questions, though daunting, can lead us to profound personal growth and spiritual development. Cancer can become a catalyst for a journey inward, where we seek to connect with our inner selves, our values, and our spirituality.

In my own journey, I discovered that healing goes far beyond the physical. While medical treatments are essential, true healing encompasses the mind, body, and spirit. This holistic approach recognizes that our emotional and spiritual

well-being are intricately connected to our physical health. Through meditation, mindfulness, and spiritual practices, I found a deeper sense of peace and resilience. I learned to listen to my body, to honor its needs, and to trust in its capacity to heal.

Cancer also has the profound ability to strengthen our relationships. When faced with such a monumental challenge, we often lean on our loved ones for support. This shared experience can bring us closer together, fostering deeper connections and a greater appreciation for the people in our lives. The support of family, friends, and even strangers becomes a lifeline, reminding us that we are not alone in our struggle. These relationships can become a source of immense strength and comfort, providing the emotional sustenance needed to navigate the difficult journey of cancer.

Moreover, cancer teaches us about resilience and the power of the human spirit. The journey through cancer is fraught with obstacles and setbacks, but it also reveals our capacity for courage, determination, and hope. Each day becomes a testament to our inner strength, as we face our fears and continue to move forward despite the uncertainty. This resilience is not just about enduring the physical aspects of the disease, but also about maintaining a positive outlook and finding joy in the small moments. It is about celebrating each victory, no matter how small, and holding on to hope even in the darkest times.

One of the most profound lessons cancer teaches us is about the importance of self-care and self-love. In our busy lives, we often neglect our own needs, prioritizing the demands of work, family, and societal expectations. Cancer forces us to slow down and pay attention to our bodies and minds. It encourages us to nurture ourselves, to listen to our inner voice, and to prioritize our well-being. This journey of self-care and self-love is not just about physical health, but also about emotional and spiritual nourishment.

In reflecting on my own experience, I have come to see cancer as a transformative force. It is an unexpected teacher that, despite its harsh methods, imparts invaluable lessons about life, love, and the human spirit. While I would never wish this journey upon anyone, I am profoundly grateful for the growth and insights it has brought into my life. Cancer has taught me to live with intention, to embrace my vulnerabilities, and to find strength in my deepest fears. It has shown me the importance of community, the power of resilience, and the beauty of the human spirit.

As you read this book, my hope is that you too will find a sense of purpose in the face of adversity. Whether you are battling cancer yourself, supporting a loved one through their journey, or simply seeking a deeper understanding of life's challenges, I invite you to look beyond the surface and explore the profound lessons that cancer can offer. Let this book be a guide, a companion, and a source of inspiration as you navigate your own path.

Cancer, in its own paradoxical way, can become a beacon of light in the darkest times. It challenges us to grow, to heal, and to transform. It reminds us of our inherent power to overcome obstacles and to find meaning in our struggles. Through this book, I hope to share the insights and wisdom I have gained, and to inspire you to discover the transformative touch of cancer on your own existence. Together, let us embrace the journey, with all its hardships and triumphs, and find the strength, healing, and purpose that lies within.

" One day you will tell your story of how you overcame what you went through ,and it will be someone else's survival guide "

Brene Brown

2

Triumph and Transformation

Growing up in the vibrant and culturally rich island of Trinidad, I had dreams that stretched far beyond its shores. At the age of twenty-four, I achieved one of those dreams by becoming a pharmacist. My path took an exciting turn when, at twenty-seven, I opened my own pharmacy with the help of a loan from my supportive father. Despite my lack of formal business education, I was determined to succeed, learning through trial and error, and drawing inspiration from my father, a highly accomplished businessman.

Opening my pharmacy in 1981 was a monumental achievement. The business quickly became successful, attracting a loyal customer base. However, my journey was not without its challenges. In 1990, a political uprising shook the country, and my pharmacy was looted. Despite the devastation, I persevered, rebuilding from the remains of my dispensary.

With the unwavering support of my customers, I not only restored my pharmacy but made it better than ever.

Located in a bustling town with a high crime rate, my pharmacy faced numerous hold-ups at gunpoint. These incidents became a grim routine, yet I pressed on, driven by my passion for serving my community. But the most harrowing ordeal came when I was kidnapped at gunpoint. The kidnapper, under the influence of drugs, forced me to drive my car, eventually putting me in the trunk. He drove us to the edge of a precipice, threatening to kill me. Strangely, in that moment of terror, I felt an overwhelming sense of peace and calm, hearing an inner voice assure me that everything would be okay.

Miraculously, the kidnapper suddenly stopped, telling me to get back in the trunk. Later, I learned that he had experienced a moment of divine intervention. The police eventually tracked him down in the hospital, and he was jailed. During the trial, I recognized him as a young man who had frequented my pharmacy. In a moment of compassion, I spoke with him, and he promised to change his life. So

I decided to give him a second chance at life .Years later, I saw the evidence of his transformation—he was married, had children, and had overcome his addiction.

Despite increasing security, the robberies continued, leaving me weary and uncomfortable. My only daughter had moved to Florida for her studies and decided to stay there. She encouraged me to join her, and in 2010, I made the life-changing decision to move to Florida. I obtained my Green Card, sold my home and pharmacy, and embarked on a new chapter in my life.

Moving to Florida was both exhilarating and daunting. With

few friends or family, I embraced the challenge, finding solace in the safety and tranquility of my new environment. My personal life also underwent significant changes. I divorced after a challenging marriage, marking the beginning of my journey toward self-discovery and healing.

In Florida, I opened a new business franchise in Naples, running it successfully for seven years before selling it just before the pandemic in 2020. During this period, I met a charming older Italian-American man in 2012, and we shared a passionate and fulfilling relationship. Though it ended in 2017, leaving me heartbroken, it also pushed me toward deeper introspection and personal growth.

Determined to find meaning in my experiences, I immersed myself in personal development. I discovered transformative teachers like Joe Vitale , Joe Dispenza,Gregg Braden, Bruce Lipton and John Assaraf , whose insights and guidance helped me navigate my inner journey. I also explored single-family real estate investing, adding another dimension to my entrepreneurial spirit.

Each experience, whether triumphant or challenging, contributed to my growth. My journey from Trinidad to Florida, from pharmacist to entrepreneur, and from fear to fearlessness, taught me invaluable lessons about resilience, compassion, and the power of inner peace. It is through these trials and tribulations that I found my true self, and it is my hope that sharing this story will inspire others to find strength and purpose in their own journeys.

My journey into understanding the deeper teachings of life had just begun to take a new and profound shift. Throughout my life, I had many spiritual awakenings, even as a child. I experienced astral traveling, receiving messages, and having out-of-body experiences during the moments between sleep and wakefulness. These experiences were mysterious and fascinating, hinting at a reality beyond the physical world.

One particularly transformative event occurred on October 31, 2016. As I was drifting off to sleep, I was suddenly enveloped by a profound and vivid humming noise. In this state, I saw a divine figure emerging from under the water, floating on a plank. The figure was clothed in a long white gown, with its back facing me. As it rose from the ocean, it began to turn around, and just as it was about to face me, a bright white light emanated from it. I knew in my heart that I was witnessing a moment of pure divinity.

This vision left an indelible mark on my soul. Even now, I can recall every detail with clarity and awe. This divine encounter was not just a fleeting dream but a powerful message, a reminder of the profound spiritual realities that exist beyond our everyday lives. It was a catalyst for my deeper exploration into spirituality and self-awareness, guiding me to seek greater understanding and connection with the divine.

3

Discovering Cancer

Discovering Cancer

In January 2017, I was caught in a whirlwind of emotional turmoil. The breakup of a six-year relationship had left me feeling like my entire world was collapsing. Hurt and despair consumed me, and I struggled to get over the heartache. Despite having experienced breakups before, this one was particularly devastating. To find solace, I turned to self-help books and discovered one on "Letting Go," which provided some much-needed guidance. Mustering all my strength and courage, I tried to move forward with my life. I filled my days with entertaining friends and clubbing, trying to mask the pain.

By May 2017, I began noticing alarming changes in my body. I couldn't control my bladder and would often find myself unable to make it to the bathroom in time. Initially, I thought it might be an infection, but since there was no burning or pain,

I dismissed it. Soon, I developed a preference for carbonated water and club sodas, accompanied by persistent stomach discomfort that felt like indigestion. I relied on antacids for temporary relief, but as weeks went by, the symptoms persisted.

Realizing something was seriously wrong, I decided to see my gynecologist. During an ultrasound, the technician casually mentioned she couldn't find my left ovary. This led to an MRI and a CA125 blood test. My doctor referred me to a gynecologic oncologist, reassuring me it was probably just a benign tumor. I clung to that hope, unable to fathom the possibility of having ovarian cancer. In denial, I turned to home remedies and natural treatments, even drinking baking soda until I felt nauseated, and extending my daily meditation sessions.

The oncologist recommended surgery for the following week, explaining that the true nature of the tumor would only be known during the operation. Staying calm, I convinced myself the surgery would be routine and that everything would be fine afterward.

On the morning of the surgery, a setback with my insurance caused a delay, forcing me to pay out of pocket. After a stressful wait, I was finally admitted to the pre operation room where I was prepped for the big procedure . The hospital staff were kind and did their best to make me comfortable, and I was grateful for the support of my daughter and sister. As I drifted into unconsciousness from the anesthetic, I had no idea how drastically my life was about to change.

Waking up from surgery, I was groggy and disoriented. Through the haze, I saw my doctor waving his hand in front of my face. His words, "We had to remove everything because your left ovary was riddled with a cancerous tumor 13 cm long," hit me like a sledgehammer. My heart sank. I had always believed cancer was something that happened to other people, not me. I lived a healthy lifestyle, eating organic foods, using natural products, and maintaining a positive mindset. Yet here I was, confronted with the harsh reality of cancer.

That evening, the effects of the anesthesia wore off, leaving me dizzy and drowsy. Hungry after over 24 hours without food, I was dismayed when my meal arrived: an overcooked steak, a dry baked potato, sweetened apple juice, and jello. The lack of nutritious options in the hospital's meal plan was appalling.

The following days in the hospital were challenging. I was heavily medicated with narcotic painkillers that caused severe constipation. My daughter's boyfriend recommended magnesium citrate, which provided relief. After a few weeks of recovery at home, I started feeling better. During a follow-up visit, my oncologist informed me that my cancer was at Stage 1. This was a huge relief, as it meant the cancer had been caught early.

Despite the relatively early stage of my cancer, my doctor advised six rounds of chemotherapy as a precaution. Although he mentioned it wasn't absolutely necessary, he strongly recommended it. My family pressured me to proceed, and, reluctantly, I agreed. In retrospect, I regretted the decision to undergo chemotherapy, feeling that it was akin to poisoning my body. Knowing what I know now, I would have chosen a different path.

My chemotherapy journey began in July. I was scheduled for six treatments, one every three weeks. The first session was a nightmare. The nurses struggled to find a suitable vein, using a vein finder machine to no avail. Eventually, the head nurse succeeded, and the infusion began. Fortunately, my sister was there to support me, and I was grateful for my family's presence during such a difficult time.

Family support became crucial in my healing journey. My four sisters took turns leaving their families to be with me during my chemotherapy treatments. Their dedication and love were invaluable, and I was eternally grateful for their unwavering support.

Two days after my first chemotherapy session, I felt extremely tired and listless. I experienced tingling in my feet and joint pain in my legs, which subsided after a few days. I focused on drinking green juices daily, prepared with the help of my sisters. Using my Omega 3 Juicer, I made nutrient-rich juices to aid in cell repair from the chemo.

The second chemotherapy session mirrored the first, with difficulties finding veins. Consequently, I had a port installed in my chest, making the process much easier. However, the side effects intensified, with increased bone pain, numbness, and tingling in my feet. When my hair began to fall out after the second treatment, I decided to shave it off entirely. Owning a franchise hair salon in Naples, I had one of my stylists buzz my head to a zero. Equipped with a wig and chemo head scarves, I faced my hairless months with a new look.

Throughout this ordeal, I questioned why cancer had come into my life. Was it to teach me about new hairstyles, or was it a sign that I needed to change my lifestyle? I realized the latter was true, but I wasn't fully aware of how much I needed to shift my daily habits.

By the third chemotherapy session, the port in my chest made treatments smoother, but the side effects persisted. My bones ached, and the tingling and numbness in my feet worsened.Despite the numerous challenges I faced during chemotherapy, I found unexpected relief in marijuana chocolate chip cookies and CBD drops. These were introduced to me by my ex-boyfriend, and they proved to be incredibly helpful. The marijuana cookies provided a sense of relaxation and comfort that eased the mental and physical strain of my treatments. Meanwhile, the CBD drops helped manage my pain and anxiety, offering a natural alternative to conventional painkillers. These remedies became an essential part of my routine, significantly improving my overall well-being during this difficult period.

I completed my six rounds of chemotherapy by the end of October 2017. All my blood results, including the CA 125 levels, returned to normal. Overjoyed, I celebrated this milestone with a big surprise party organized by my daughter. Friends and family from all over the country, and even abroad, joined the festivities. It was a joyous occasion with a DJ and caterers, and I reveled in the celebration of having come so far in my battle against cancer.

The journey through cancer was a transformative experience. It taught me resilience, the importance of family support, and the need to listen to my body. As I continue to reflect on this chapter of my life, I am grateful for the lessons learned and the strength I discovered within myself. Through it all, I emerged with a deeper understanding of life, love, and the power of inner healing.

4

Overcoming New Challenges

Overcoming New Challenges

As time went by, I believed I was becoming stronger, more resilient, but little did I know what I was about to face. Each day felt like a small victory against the shadows of my past, yet the universe had more trials in store for me.

My skin had darkened considerably after chemotherapy, looking dry and burnt. By April 2018, it started to regain a healthier color and tone. My hair, however, was a different story. It began to grow back, but the texture was coarse, with almost bald patches on the top and sides of my head. I thought by now my hair should be back to normal, but it wasn't. I didn't want to wear wigs for the rest of my life. They were uncomfortable and looked fake.

Desperate for a solution, I found a clinic in Naples offering PRP - Plasma Rich Platelets - treatments for hair loss. Coincidentally, the doctor who owned the clinic came to my bar-bershop to introduce PRP treatments. I seized the opportunity to start treatment. After the first session, I noticed some new hair growth but nothing significant. Undeterred, I proceeded with a couple more treatments, but they yielded no noticeable difference. Money wasted with no results.

My new hair growth was now almost entirely gray. Embrac-ing the change, I decided to purchase new salt-and-pepper wigs, with more salt than pepper. Surprisingly, they looked quite nice, and I received many compliments. One memorable encounter was with a neighbor in Costco. She hailed me from a distance, and when I didn't recognize her at first, she approached me and said, "I love your hair color. I've wanted to go natural as I'm getting older but didn't have the courage. You look great and give me the courage to go natural!"

Little did she know I was sporting a wig!

Her comment took me aback, reminding me how our mere presence can impact others' lives in profound ways.

In early 2018, I traveled to Maui with my daughter and other family members. We had a fantastic time with my soon-to-be son-in-law, partying hard, attending a luau, dining at fancy restaurants, and relaxing on beautiful beaches. We even went on a submarine tour, which was a lot of fun. Our adventure continued with a few days in Hollywood, driving through Beverly Hills and Rodeo Drive, catching glimpses of homes where movie stars lived. I indulged in many glasses of wine and beer, thinking this was my first real holiday after the stressful ordeal with cancer. But was I doing the right thing? Was I heading down the same beaten path?

Life felt good. My orchids were in full bloom, looking alive and healthy, making me feel like I was also blooming. Then, life took another unexpected turn. One morning, as I was changing clothes, I noticed a big protrusion in my belly, on the side where I had the incision from my major surgery in 2017. Panic set in. What was happening? It felt like a hernia, with my intestines protruding against the incision site. My oncologist dismissed it as just a hernia and referred me to a general surgeon for repair. He didn't mention it was an incisional hernia resulting from the previous surgery.

The surgeon in Naples suggested using a "safe" mesh to repair the hernia, cutting along the same vertical incision. I asked about alternatives to mesh, but he assured me the new mesh was safe, and any surgeon would likely offer the same option. Reluctantly, I agreed to the mesh repair, despite my reservations.

In April 2018, exactly a year after my first surgery, I underwent my second surgery. The procedure involved staples and a drain bag, similar to my first surgery. My belly felt heavy and uncomfortable, and I had to avoid lifting anything heavy to prevent complications. Reflecting on it now, I wish I had paid out-of-pocket for the non-mesh hernia repair. It might have yielded better results, but I didn't know better at the time.

Determined to regain my strength, I took another short vacation to Reno, Nevada, and spent two lovely days at Lake Tahoe, enjoying the beautiful views. As time approached for my dream adventure to Europe, I felt strong and healthy, ready for a big journey.

In September 2018, I embarked on a Western Mediterranean cruise on a Celebrity Ship, starting in Barcelona. The architecture and food in Barcelona were amazing. From there, we visited Spain's Valencia and Granada, Gibraltar, the South of France's Cannes and Nice, and Italy's Rome and Amalfi

Coast before returning to Barcelona. I went with my family and had a blast. We took numerous tours and did plenty of walking. Despite the physical exertion, I managed to cope with all the activities. Onboard, we ate, drank, danced, and laughed, enjoying many fun nights.

Upon returning, I felt a strong urge to seek a deeper meaning in life. Why had cancer come my way? What was I supposed to learn? I believed events in our lives happen for a purpose, not by mere coincidence. My search led me to Dr. Sue Morter and the Energy Codes. I was always fascinated by the idea that we are energy beings and resonated with the five main reasons for Creation according to Bashar:

1. We exist.
2. All is one and one is all.
3. Everything is here and now.
4. What you put out is what you get back.
5. Change is the only constant in life; everything changes except the first four laws.

I knew these laws as a teenager. I don't know how, but I did. I used to look up at the sky for inspiration, and ideas just came to me. We all have the ability to connect with the universe deeply; we just need to be receptive, open, and in tune with its rhythm.

I signed up for a course to become an Energy Codes Facilitator with Dr. Sue Morter. I learned so much about being an energetic being of light, different breathing techniques, and more. She opened my eyes and heart to a new way of existing. The course lasted a few months, culminating in a meeting with Dr. Sue in Los Angeles in March 2019, where I received my certificate. I felt like a new, awakened being.

I also pursued a course with Marisa Peer from Mind Valley on hypnosis. Earlier in my life, I had learned from Joe Vitale and Steve G. Jones, which was quite helpful and informative. I believe in continuous learning and personal development, always expanding my mind as far as possible.

I continued trying to eat healthy, though I occasionally strayed to comfort foods from my past. I was overjoyed when my daughter got pregnant after trying for some time. Then disaster struck again.

In August 2019, I woke up with severe abdominal pain. At first, I thought it was gas pain or constipation. The pain was gripping, and I felt feverish. Suspecting an infection, I called my sister, who lived nearby. She rushed me to the Emergency Room at Lee Health in Coconut Point. Admitted immediately, I met a kind doctor who ran several tests. As I suspected, it was a severe case of diverticulitis. He insisted on hospitalization for IV antibiotic treatment, warning that my colon could rupture otherwise.

Reluctantly, I agreed and was transported by ambulance to Health Park Hospital in Fort Myers. It was my first ambulance ride and experience as a patient on a stretcher. The ride was smooth, and the pain subsided somewhat with medication. Upon arrival, I was taken straight to the ward, bypassing the lengthy admission process, which I appreciated.

I spent four days at the hospital, receiving IV antibiotics, drips, and undergoing various tests, including a colonoscopy. The nurses struggled to find my veins since my port had been removed a year after my cancer surgery. Those were long, dreary days, but I finally felt better and was able to return home.

Reflecting on my diet and lifestyle, I began to wonder if these habits were contributing to my ongoing health issues or if they were lingering consequences of my ovarian cancer treatment or the mesh implant from my hernia repair. This introspection led to a realization that perhaps my body was reacting to the accumulated stress and dietary choices I had made over the years. I started to question every aspect of my daily routine: the foods I ate, the level of physical activity I engaged in, and even the ways I managed stress. Was my frequent indulgence in comfort foods exacerbating my problems? Were the occasional processed foods and junk food weakening my immune system and making me more susceptible to health issues?

Determined to take control of my health and ensure my body received the care it deserved, I embarked on a comprehensive journey to find answers. This journey was not just about seeking medical opinions but also about delving deep into holistic health practices. I began researching various dietary plans, from plant-based diets to ketogenic and Mediterranean diets, trying to understand which could best support my recovery and long-term health. I read countless books and articles, attended health seminars, and consulted with nutritionists and holistic health practitioners.

In addition to dietary changes, I explored different forms of exercise that could strengthen my body without putting undue strain on my recovering muscles and joints. Yoga, Pilates, and gentle strength training became integral parts of my daily routine. I also incorporated mindfulness practices such as meditation and deep breathing exercises to help manage stress and improve my mental well-being.

My journey also included experimenting with various

supplements and natural remedies known for their healing properties. I discovered the benefits of probiotics for gut health, omega-3 fatty acids for reducing inflammation, and antioxidant-rich foods for boosting my immune system.

Throughout this process, I documented my experiences, noting what worked and what didn't, making adjustments as needed. This journey was not easy; it required patience, perseverance, and a willingness to continuously learn and adapt. However, each small step forward brought me closer to a healthier, more balanced life.

This quest for better health was also a journey of self-discovery. I learned to listen to my body, understanding its signals and responding to its needs. I realized the importance of self-care and the power of positive thinking in the healing process. By taking charge of my health, I found a renewed sense of purpose and a deeper appreciation for life.

In the end, this journey was about more than just physical health. It was about finding a holistic approach to wellness that nurtured my body, mind, and spirit. It was about building a lifestyle that supported my overall well-being, allowing me to live a vibrant, fulfilling life despite the challenges I faced.

5

Healing - Trying Different Modalities

Healing - Trying Different Modalities

My journey to healing began with a deep, determined search for answers. I knew I couldn't continue with the same lifestyle, as it might lead to a recurrence of the cancer. As Albert Einstein once stated, "Insanity is doing the same thing over and over again and expecting different results." I was on a mission to find a better way of being.

I fervently searched the internet until I discovered Functional Medicine. Having followed conventional medicine for most of my life as a pharmacist, this new approach to medicine made much more sense to me. I began to understand that our bodies are incredibly intelligent and have the ability to heal themselves with a positive mindset, a suitable environment, and total awareness of the present moment. One of my mentors, Sachin Patel, summed it up perfectly: "The Doctor of the future is the Patient!"

As I delved deeper into this new way of thinking, I came across Dr. Mark Hyman and Dr. Jeffrey Bland, who introduced me to the concept of getting to the root cause of an ailment or disease rather than just treating the symptoms. Conventional medicine often focuses on symptom management, but Functional Medicine looks at the bigger picture.

One morning, while scrolling on Facebook, I came across a course from the Functional Nutrition Alliance taught by Andrea Nakayama. It offered certification as a Functional Nutrition Counselor, and I immediately registered and got started. The course was intense, requiring long hours of study, but my background in human biology as a pharmacist made it easier to grasp and retain the information.

I began with "The Good Riddance" program, a four-week regimen designed to shift my diet and lifestyle. The program was gluten, dairy, and sugar-free and came with a well-laid-out recipe guide. Following this protocol, I noticed significant changes. My scalp, which had been plagued by psoriasis since my teenage years, stopped itching. I had tried numerous treatments from dermatologists, but none had cured the condition. To my amazement, avoiding gluten healed my psoriasis, which had always been considered an autoimmune disease with no cure.

Here is some information I gathered about gluten:

Why Eating Gluten in the USA Can Be Harmful to the Gut and Overall Health

The Nature of Gluten

Gluten is a protein found in wheat, barley, and rye. It gives dough its elasticity and helps it rise and maintain its shape. While gluten itself isn't inherently harmful to most people, its effects can vary greatly depending on individual sensitivities, the quantity consumed, and the quality of the gluten-containing foods.

Gluten Sensitivity and Celiac Disease

For some people, eating gluten can cause serious health issues:

Celiac Disease:

This autoimmune disorder affects about 1% of the population. When people with celiac disease consume gluten, their immune system attacks the lining of their small intestine. This can lead to severe nutritional deficiencies, gastrointestinal issues, and a host of other symptoms, including fatigue, anemia, and joint pain.

Non-Celiac Gluten Sensitivity (NCGS):

Some individuals experience symptoms similar to celiac disease without the autoimmune response or intestinal damage. Symptoms of NCGS can include bloating, diarrhea, abdominal pain, and fatigue.

The State of Wheat in the USA

**Hybridization and Genetic Modification: Over the decades, wheat in the USA has undergone significant changes through hybridization to increase yields and resistance to pests. This modern wheat, often referred to as "dwarf wheat," contains higher levels of gluten and other proteins that can be more difficult for some people to digest compared to ancient grains like einkorn or emmer.

Glyphosate Use:

Glyphosate, a common herbicide known by the brand name Roundup, is often used on wheat crops in the USA. It is applied to help dry the crops before harvest, a process known as desiccation. Residues of glyphosate have been found in wheat products, raising concerns about its impact on human health, particularly gut health. Glyphosate is suspected to act as an antibiotic in the gut, disrupting the balance of beneficial bacteria.

Processing Methods:

Many gluten-containing foods in the USA are highly processed. Refined wheat products such as white bread, pastries, and other baked goods often contain additives, preservatives, and high levels of sugar, which can further irritate the gut and contribute to inflammation.

Impact on Gut Health

Leaky Gut Syndrome: Gluten can increase intestinal permeability in some people. This condition, often referred to as "leaky gut," allows undigested food particles, toxins, and microbes to leak into the bloodstream, potentially triggering widespread inflammation and an immune response.

Microbiome Disruption:

The gut microbiome plays a crucial role in digestion, immune function, and overall health. Gluten and glyphosate exposure can disrupt the balance of gut bacteria, leading to dysbiosis (an imbalance in the gut microbiome). Dysbiosis has been linked to numerous health issues, including inflammatory bowel disease (IBD), irritable bowel syndrome (IBS), and even mental health conditions like anxiety and depression.

Chronic Inflammation:

Gluten can trigger inflammatory responses in susceptible individuals. Chronic inflammation is a key factor in many modern chronic diseases, including heart disease, diabetes, and certain types of cancer.

Conclusion

While gluten itself is not inherently harmful to everyone, its effects can be particularly pronounced in the USA due to the high gluten content of modern wheat, the use of glyphosate, and the prevalence of highly processed foods. These factors can contribute to gut health issues and broader health concerns.

In 2022 I had a DNA test which gave very comprehensive reports and sure enough , I have a sensitivity to Gluten and Dairy , so I try to avoid them .

After the four weeks were over, I continued with the same diet and felt incredibly good. My joint pains disappeared, and my finger joints, which had become enlarged and misshapen, started returning to normal. I was elated and happy to experience this "new" me. I continued learning and eventually excelled in the final exam, achieving a passing grade of 100 percent. I felt accomplished and awakened to a new reality, eager to help others struggling with similar issues.

I also observed weight loss, especially around my waist and abdomen. Knowing I was on the right track, I wondered how I could share my knowledge with others, particularly menopausal women like myself. The answer came again while scrolling on Facebook. In April 2021, I saw an advertisement for a course from Perfect Practice, hosted by Dr. Sachin Patel. It appealed to me as it promised to teach how to set up an online practice to help clients balance their blood sugar, hormones, and lose weight through lifestyle shifts.

I enrolled in the course, which was expensive but well worth it. I stayed with the program for two years, setting up my website and producing an online course. I hosted numerous webinars, marketed my program extensively, and enrolled many women in a six-week intensive lifestyle shift program.

However, while deepening my involvement in nutrition, I faced another challenge. I noticed a shift in my bowel patterns, with gas that smells like rotten eggs, indicating hydrogen sulfide. As a practitioner, I decided to test for Small Intestinal Bacterial Overgrowth (SIBO), which revealed high levels of methane gas. Realizing I had a leaky gut, I sought help from a Functional Medicine practitioner.

I found Dr. Lindsey Berkson in Naples, who was amazing. We worked together to manage my SIBO. Preferring to avoid conventional antibiotics, I opted for herbal treatments.

Here is some information I gathered about SIBO:

Understanding SIBO and Its Natural Treatments

What is SIBO?

Small Intestinal Bacterial Overgrowth (SIBO) is a condition where an excessive amount of bacteria is present in the small intestine. Unlike the large intestine, which is designed to host a large population of bacteria, the small intestine should have relatively few. The overgrowth of bacteria in the small intestine can lead to various gastrointestinal symptoms and nutritional deficiencies.

Symptoms of SIBO

- Bloating
- Abdominal pain or discomfort

- Diarrhea or constipation
- Gas and belching
- Malabsorption of nutrients, leading to deficiencies
- Weight loss or weight gain
- Fatigue
- Nausea

Causes of SIBO

SIBO can be caused by a variety of factors that affect the normal movement and function of the small intestine, including:

- Impaired motility:

Conditions such as irritable bowel syndrome (IBS), diabetes, and scleroderma can slow down the motility of the small intestine.

- Structural abnormalities:

Surgery or conditions like Crohn's disease can create pockets or obstructions in the intestine where bacteria can overgrow.

- Immune system issues:

A weakened immune system can fail to control the bacterial population in the small intestine.

- Medications:

Long-term use of antibiotics, proton pump inhibitors (PPIs), and other medications can disrupt the balance of gut bacteria.

Natural Treatments for SIBO

Dietary Changes:

-Low FODMAP Diet: This diet involves avoiding certain carbohydrates that are poorly absorbed and easily fermented by bacteria, such as certain fruits, vegetables, grains, and dairy products. This diet helps reduce the food supply for bacteria in the small intestine.

- Specific Carbohydrate Diet (SCD):
Similar to the low FODMAP diet, the SCD restricts complex carbohydrates to starve the overgrown bacteria.

- Elemental Diet:
This is a liquid diet composed of easily digestible nutrients. It can be used for a short period to reduce bacterial load by starving the bacteria of fermentable carbohydrates.

Herbal Antibiotics:
Several herbal remedies have been found effective in treating SIBO by reducing bacterial overgrowth:

- Oregano oil:Contains carvacrol and thymol, which have strong antimicrobial properties.

- Berberine: Found in herbs like goldenseal, barberry, and Oregon grape, berberine has broad-spectrum antimicrobial effects.

- Neem: Known for its antibacterial and anti-inflammatory properties.

- Garlic extract: Contains allicin, which has antibacterial properties.

Probiotics:
Probiotics can help restore a healthy balance of gut bacteria. Specific strains, such as Saccharomyces boulardii and Lactobacillus species, have been shown to be particularly beneficial for SIBO.

Digestive Support:
- Digestive enzymes: Supplementing with digestive enzymes can help break down food more efficiently, reducing the amount of undigested food available for bacterial fermentation.

- Betaine HCl:
For individuals with low stomach acid, supplementing with

Betaine HCl can improve digestion and prevent bacterial overgrowth.

Lifestyle Modifications:

- Meal spacing: Eating smaller, more frequent meals can help improve intestinal motility and reduce the chance of bacterial overgrowth.

- Stress management:Stress can impact gut health. Practices such as yoga, meditation, and mindfulness can help reduce stress levels.

-Exercise: Regular physical activity can enhance gut motility and overall digestive health.

Gut Motility Agents:

Natural agents that support gut motility, such as ginger and iberis amara , can be helpful in promoting the normal movement of the small intestine, thereby preventing bacterial overgrowth.

Monitoring and Maintenance

After initial treatment, it is important to maintain the balance of gut bacteria to prevent recurrence. This can involve:

- Continued dietary management
- Regular use of probiotics
- Periodic use of herbal antimicrobials if symptoms return
- Ongoing stress management and lifestyle adjustments

Conclusion

SIBO is a challenging condition that can significantly impact quality of life. However, through a combination of dietary changes, herbal remedies, probiotics, digestive support, and lifestyle modifications, it is possible to manage SIBO naturally and effectively.

I am just writing this for your general information .

(Always consult with a healthcare professional before starting any new treatment to ensure it is appropriate for your individual health needs.)

I listened to Dr Tom O'Brien and tried Colostrum and HMO (Human Milk Oligosaccharide) for Gut repair . Also tried Pectasol from Dr Isaac Eliaz.

These products worked as an adjunct to my healing gut protocol .

I chose the herbal route, using oregano oil capsules, berberine, garlic, probiotics, digestive enzymes, and Betaine HCl for several months. I also took high doses of Omega-3 fish oil and SPM Active to reduce gut inflammation. Over time, my SIBO symptoms diminished, and my gut health improved.

My functional medicine doctor prescribed low-dose Naltrexone, melatonin, and high-dose vitamin C to prevent tumor growth, along with Iodoral to reduce the risk of breast cancer. Additional supplements included Vitamin D3 + K2, Vitamin B Complex, multivitamins, quercetin, magnesium, zinc, milk thistle, resveratrol, tocotrienols,fiber,probiotics, digestive enzymes and tributyrin. I continue to use these supplements today.

Due to the removal of my ovaries and being post menopausal , I also faced hormonal imbalances. My doctor prescribed Bioidentical Hormone Replacement Therapy (BHRT), initially administered vaginally and now topically. Most conventional doctors are skeptical about prescribing BHRT, especially for someone with a history of ovarian cancer. However, BHRT has been incredibly beneficial for me.

Here is some information I gathered on why BHRT is beneficial:

Bioidentical Hormone Replacement Therapy (BHRT) can be particularly beneficial for postmenopausal women who have had their ovaries and reproductive system completely removed due to Stage 1 ovarian cancer. Here's why:

Hormone Balance Restoration

Hormone Deficiency Post-Surgery: The removal of ovaries and the reproductive system results in an abrupt halt in the production of key hormones such as estrogen, progesterone, and testosterone. This sudden hormonal imbalance can lead to severe menopausal symptoms.

Alleviating Menopausal Symptoms:

BHRT helps replenish the body's hormone levels with compounds that are chemically identical to those produced naturally. This can significantly reduce symptoms such as hot flashes, night sweats, vaginal dryness, mood swings, and sleep disturbances, improving overall quality of life.

Bone Health

Preventing Osteoporosis:Estrogen plays a crucial role in maintaining bone density. After the removal of ovaries, the risk of osteoporosis increases due to decreased estrogen levels. BHRT can help maintain bone density and reduce the risk of fractures and osteoporosis.

Cardiovascular Health

Cardiovascular Protection: Estrogen has protective effects on the cardiovascular system. Postmenopausal women with low estrogen levels have a higher risk of developing cardiovascular diseases. BHRT can help in maintaining heart health by improving lipid profiles and vascular function.

Cognitive Function

Improving Cognitive Function: Hormone deficiencies can affect cognitive functions, leading to memory issues and difficulty concentrating. BHRT may help in preserving cognitive function and reducing the risk of neurodegenerative diseases.

Emotional and Psychological Well-being

Enhancing Mood and Emotional Stability: Hormonal imbalances can lead to mood swings, depression, and anxiety. BHRT can help stabilize hormone levels, thereby improving mood and emotional well-being.

Personalized Treatment

Customized to Individual Needs: BHRT is often tailored to the individual's specific hormonal needs, ensuring a more personalized approach to hormone replacement. This customization can optimize the therapeutic effects and minimize potential side effects.

Safety Considerations

Monitoring and Adjustments:Regular monitoring and appropriate adjustments by a healthcare provider ensure that BHRT remains safe and effective. It's important for women with a history of cancer to have their hormone levels and overall health regularly assessed.

In conclusion,

BHRT can offer significant benefits for postmenopausal women who have undergone surgical removal of their ovaries and reproductive system due to ovarian cancer. By restoring hormonal balance, BHRT can alleviate menopausal symptoms, protect bone and cardiovascular health, enhance cognitive function, and improve overall emotional well-being, leading to a better quality of life.

(However, it is essential to consult with a healthcare provider to ensure the therapy is appropriate and tailored to individual health needs).

BHRT helped restore my hormonal balance, alleviating severe menopausal symptoms. My previous bone density tests (Dexa Scan) showed osteoporosis in my left hip and osteopenia in my lower spine. To my delight, my most recent Dexa Scan showed vast improvement in my bone density after one year of BHRT treatment, which I attribute to this therapy.

Overall, my journey through various healing modalities has been transformative. From diet changes to functional medicine, herbal treatments, and BHRT, each step has brought me closer to a healthier, more balanced life. This experience has empowered me to share my knowledge and help others on their healing journeys.

I am still on my journey to being as healthy as I possibly can , so I keep updated with some of the latest research . I listen to many health podcasts, especially those by Ari Whiten and some bio hacking information from Nathalie Niddam on peptides . I even tried using Methylene Blue to improve mitochondrial function . I still use it to this day . I take it for a few weeks then stop and repeat .

I even invested in an Infrared sauna in 2019 ,which I placed in my garage . I try to use it at least three times a week for at least thirty minutes at 140 degrees Fahrenheit .

Must perform dry brushing before the sauna as it stimulates the Lymphatic System

Here are some of the benefits of using an Infrared Sauna

The Benefits of Infrared Sauna

Infrared saunas offer a range of health benefits that go beyond traditional saunas. The infrared heat penetrates deeply into the body, promoting relaxation, detoxification, and overall well-being. Key benefits include:

Detoxification:

Sweating helps eliminate toxins and heavy metals from the body, enhancing detoxification.

Improved Circulation:

Infrared heat boosts blood flow, supporting cardiovascular health and speeding up muscle recovery.

Pain Relief:

The deep heat alleviates joint and muscle pain, making it ideal for those with arthritis or chronic pain.

Skin Health:

Regular use can improve skin tone, reduce wrinkles, and enhance overall skin clarity.

Relaxation and Stress Relief:

The soothing warmth helps reduce stress, lower cortisol levels, and promote a sense of well-being.

If you are new to saunas, start with a lower temperature and shorter sessions. Gradually increase the temperature and duration as you become more accustomed until you reach your desired comfort level.

6

Conclusion- Transformative Changes and Life Lessons

Conclusion- Transformative Changes and Life Lessons

As I continue on my journey to wellness, I strive to engage in various activities that broaden my opportunities for healing. These endeavors often extend beyond direct health interventions to encompass my general well-being. Life is a journey filled with suffering, and it is through this suffering that we build our strength and resilience, becoming stronger in every sense—mentally, spiritually, physically, and emotionally. This newfound strength equips us to face future challenges with greater fortitude.

The Catalyst for Change

One of the most significant ways cancer can be a blessing is by acting as a powerful catalyst for change. Before my diagnosis, I was caught in the whirlwind of everyday life, often ignoring the subtle signs my body was giving me. The diagnosis forced me to stop, reflect, and reassess my priorities. It was a wake-up call that prompted me to make essential changes in my lifestyle, diet, and overall approach to health. The realization that I could no longer take my health for granted spurred me to adopt healthier habits, seek out new forms of healing, and explore alternative medicine.

A poignant moment in my journey came when my granddaughter was born prematurely, facing her own set of challenges. In that vulnerable time, I made a promise to myself and the Universe: I would be there for her for as long as possible. This promise became a powerful catalyst for me to live a healthier life. One of the most significant changes I made was deciding to stop drinking all forms of alcohol. My granddaughter became my biggest inspiration, giving me a profound reason to pursue a healthier lifestyle. Today, I am grateful for that decision, as I feel and look better for it.

Appreciation for Life

Cancer brings an acute awareness of mortality, which, paradoxically, can lead to a deeper appreciation for life. The knowledge that life is finite encourages us to savor each moment, cherish our relationships, and focus on what truly matters. It strips away the superficial layers, leaving us with a raw, unfiltered perspective on life. This newfound appreciation can enhance our daily experiences, making us more grateful for the simple joys and more resilient in the face of challenges.It truly allows us to feel and know that we are all part of the Divine Consciousness made of pure Love and Light !

Strength and Resilience

Going through cancer treatment is undoubtedly one of the most physically and emotionally challenging experiences a person can endure. However, it is precisely through these hardships that we discover our inner strength and resilience. The journey through cancer is a testament to human fortitude. Each day becomes a battle won, each small victory a reason to celebrate. This resilience extends beyond the illness, equipping us with the tools to face future adversities with greater confidence and determination.

Deeper Connections

Cancer has a unique way of bringing people together. The outpouring of support from family, friends, and even strangers can be overwhelming and profoundly touching. This experience fosters deeper connections and strengthens bonds that might have otherwise remained superficial. It teaches us the importance of leaning on others, of accepting help, and of being there for one another. These strengthened relationships can become a source of immense comfort and support, not just during the illness but throughout life.

Spiritual Awakening

For many, a cancer diagnosis can trigger a spiritual awakening. The confrontation with one's mortality often leads to a quest for deeper meaning and purpose. This journey can take many forms, from exploring different spiritual practices to finding solace in nature, art, or meditation. My own journey led me to explore functional medicine and holistic healing, which opened my eyes to the interconnectedness of mind, body, and spirit. This spiritual awakening can bring a profound sense of peace, purpose, and connection to something greater than oneself.

I developed a deep appreciation for Dr. Joe Dispenza's teachings and became an advanced student, eagerly attending his workshops and weeklong events. Immersing myself in his methodology, I began practicing his meditations regularly and found them incredibly enlightening. Through these meditative practices, I became more attuned to the Universe, which opened the door to profound spiritual experiences. I felt a deep connection with the Divine, experiencing moments of intense clarity and insight that transcended ordinary understanding. These experiences not only enriched my spiritual life but also reinforced my belief in the interconnectedness of mind, body, and spirit, guiding me toward a deeper sense of peace and purpose.

I had the privilege of training with the esteemed Dr. Tony Nader, the leader of the Transcendental Meditation (T.M.) Movement. His teachings on consciousness have played a significant role in my spiritual awakening. Integrating his insights, I frequently practice Transcendental Meditation both in the mornings and occasionally at night. These meditative sessions have become a cornerstone of my daily routine, fostering a deeper sense of awareness and inner peace.

Personal Growth and Transformation

Cancer can be a profound teacher, guiding us toward personal growth and transformation. It forces us to confront our deepest fears, question our beliefs, and reassess our goals. This introspection can lead to significant personal development, helping us become more empathetic, compassionate, and self-aware. The journey through cancer often leaves us transformed, with a deeper understanding of ourselves and a clearer sense of our place in the world.

Lessons in Self-Care

One of the most valuable lessons cancer teaches is the importance of self-care. Before my diagnosis, I often neglected my own needs, prioritizing work and other responsibilities over my well-being. Cancer forced me to put myself first, to listen to my body, and to make self-care a priority. This shift in perspective has had a lasting impact, encouraging me to adopt healthier habits, set boundaries, and make time for rest and rejuvenation.

Empowerment Through Knowledge

Navigating a cancer diagnosis often involves a steep learning curve. From understanding the disease itself to exploring treatment options and lifestyle changes, the journey is one of continuous education. This empowerment through knowledge is invaluable. It not only equips us with the tools to make informed decisions about our health but also fosters a sense of control and agency in a situation that often feels overwhelmingly uncertain.

Embracing a New Perspective

Cancer has a way of shifting our perspective, encouraging us to see the world through a different lens. The things that once seemed important may no longer hold the same significance, while previously overlooked aspects of life gain newfound importance. This shift in perspective can lead to a more balanced, fulfilling life. It encourages us to live with intention, to focus on what truly brings us joy, and to let go of the things that no longer serve us.

Advocacy and Purpose

For many cancer survivors, the journey doesn't end with remission. Instead, it marks the beginning of a new chapter, one that often involves advocacy and a renewed sense of purpose. Sharing our experiences, raising awareness, and supporting others going through similar struggles can be incredibly fulfilling. It allows us to turn our pain into purpose, to make a positive impact on the world, and to give back to the community that supported us during our journey.

Rekindling Passions and Exploring New Opportunities

In July 2022, I rekindled my passion for real estate investing by joining Grant Cardone's Mentorship Program for a year. There, I met many interesting entrepreneurs, joined various groups, and learned about syndication with multifamily apartment complexes. This new endeavor has been both challenging and rewarding, and I continue to learn and grow in this field.

In 2023, I joined Multifamily Mindset, another community of like-minded individuals passionate about real estate. Being part of these communities has been incredibly fulfilling and healthy, providing a sense of belonging and purpose.

My study partner from the Functional Nutrition program encouraged me to become an insurance agent, suggesting it would be a fun and different experience. Intrigued, I wrote the state board exams and became licensed. I now primarily focus on life, health, and annuities policies, helping educate families to secure a better financial future.

Conclusion – A Blessing in Disguise

In conclusion, while cancer is undoubtedly a formidable adversary, it also holds the potential to be a profound teacher and a catalyst for positive change. It forces us to confront our vulnerabilities, appreciate the fragility of life, and embrace the strength within us. The journey through cancer, though arduous, can lead to a richer, more meaningful existence. It can deepen our connections, foster personal growth, and guide us toward a more holistic approach to health and well-being.

Cancer teaches us to live with intention, to cherish each moment, and to seek out the lessons hidden within our struggles. It reminds us that even in the darkest times, there is potential for light and growth. By embracing these lessons, we can transform a seemingly insurmountable challenge into an opportunity for profound personal transformation. While no one wishes for cancer, those who face it can emerge stronger, wiser, and more resilient, with a deeper appreciation for the precious gift of life.

If you found this book helpful ,I'd be very appreciative if you left a favorable review for the book on Amazon .

7

References

References

Beever, R. (2009). *Far-infrared saunas for treatment of cardiovascular risk factors: Summary of published evidence. *Canadian Family Physician*, 55(7), 691-696. PMID: 19587627*

Biesiekierski, J. R., Newnham, E. D., Irving, P. M., Barrett, J. S., Haines, M., Doecke, J. D., ... & Gibson, P. R. (2011). Gluten causes gastrointestinal symptoms in subjects without celiac disease: A double-blind randomized placebo-controlled trial. *American Journal of Gastroenterology*, 106(3), 508-514. https://doi.org/10.1038/ajg.2010.487

Catassi, C., Bai, J. C., Bonaz, B., Bouma, G., Calabrò, A., Carroccio, A., ... & Fasano, A. (2013). Non-celiac gluten sensitivity: The new frontier of gluten related disorders. *Nutrients*, 5(10), 3839-3853. https://doi.org/10.3390/nu5103839

Chedid, V., Dhalla, S., Clarke, J. O., Roland, B. C., Dunbar, K. B., Koh, J. M., & Mullin, G. E. (2014). Herbal therapy is equivalent to rifaximin for the treatment of small intestinal bacterial overgrowth. *Global Advances in Health and Medicine*, 3(3), 16-24. https://doi.org/10.7453/gahmj.2014.019

Cirigliano, M. (2007). Bioidentical hormone therapy: a review of the evidence. *Journal of Women's Health*, 16(5), 600-631. https://doi.org/10.1089/jwh.2006.0174

Fasano, A., & Catassi, C. (2012). Clinical practice. Celiac disease. *New England Journal of Medicine*, 367(25), 2419-2426. https://doi.org/10.1056/NEJMcp1113994

Fitzpatrick, L. A. (2015). Estrogen therapy for postmenopausal osteoporosis. *Endocrine*, 50(2), 477-484. https://doi.org/10.1007/s12020-015-0559-2

Ghoshal, U. C., Shukla, R., & Ghoshal, U. (2017). Small intestinal bacterial overgrowth and irritable bowel syndrome: A bridge between functional organic dichotomy. *Gut and Liver*, 11(2), 196-208. https://doi.org/10.5009/gnl15521

Holtorf, K. (2009). The bioidentical hormone debate: Are bioidentical hormones (estradiol, estriol, and progesterone) safe and effective? *Postgraduate Medicine*, 121(1), 73-85. https://doi.org/10.3810/pgm.2009.01.1949

Hussain, J., & Cohen, M. (2018). Clinical effects of regular dry sauna bathing: A systematic review. *Evidence-Based Complementary and Alternative Medicine*, 2018, Article ID 1857413. https://doi.org/10.1155/2018/1857413

Kaunitz, A. M., & Manson, J. E. (2015). Management of menopausal symptoms. *Obstetrics & Gynecology*, 126(4), 859-876. https://doi.org/10.1097/AOG.0000000000001058

Lappegard, K. T., & Ronnestad, A. (2009). Effects of regular sauna bathing on chronic pain and quality of life in patients with chronic tension-type headache: A pilot study. *Journal of Psychosomatic Research*, 66(4), 389-393. https://doi.org/10.1016/j.jpsychores.2009.01.012

Maki, P. M., & Henderson, V. W. (2012). Cognitive function during the menopausal transition. *Menopause*, 19(5), 535-541. https://doi.org/10.1097/gme.0b013e31824acac1

Mero, A., Tornberg, J., & Ojala, T. (2014). Effects of far-infrared sauna bathing on recovery from strength and endurance training sessions in men. *Journal of Clinical Medicine Research*, 6(5), 329-336. https://doi.org/10.14740/jocmr1866w

Perlmutter, D., & Loberg, K. (2013). *Grain brain: The surprising truth about wheat, carbs, and sugar—Your brain's silent killers.* Little, Brown Spark. ISBN: 978-0316234801

Pinkerton, J. V., & Stovall, D. W. (2010). Reconsidering the nonhormonal management of menopause-associated vasomotor symptoms: Is it time to give these therapies another chance? *Journal of Women's Health*, 19(5), 933-948. https://doi.org/10.1089/jwh.2009.1740

Pimentel, M., Lembo, A., & Rao, S. S. (2020). A 14-day elemental diet is highly effective in normalizing the lactulose breath test. *Digestive Diseases and Sciences*, 49(1), 73-77. https://doi.org/10.1023/B:DDAS.0000011612.95652.5e

Reilly, N. R., & Green, P. H. (2012). Epidemiology and clinical presentations of celiac disease. *Seminars in Immunopathology*, 34(4), 473-478. https://doi.org/10.1007/s00281-012-0329-4

Rubio-Tapia, A., Ludvigsson, J. F., Brantner, T. L., Murray, J. A., & Everhart, J. E. (2012). The prevalence of celiac disease in the United States. *American Journal of Gastroenterology*, 107(10), 1538-1544. https://doi.org/10.1038/ajg.2012.219

Samsel, A., & Seneff, S. (2013). Glyphosate, pathways to modern diseases II: Celiac sprue and gluten intolerance. *Interdisciplinary Toxicology*, 6(4), 159-184. https://doi.org/10.2478/intox-2013-0026

Sood, R., Faubion, S. S., Kuhle, C. L., Thielen, J. M., & Shuster, L. T. (2011). Prescribing hormone therapy for menopausal symptoms: What's a clinician to do? *Mayo Clinic Proceedings*, 86(5), 494-500. https://doi.org/10.4065/mcp.2010.0717

Staudacher, H. M., & Whelan, K. (2017). The low FODMAP diet: Recent advances in understanding its mechanisms and efficacy in IBS. *Gut*, 66(8), 1517-1527. https://doi.org/10.1136/gutjnl-2017-313750

Utian, W. H., & Schiff, I. (2012). NAMS-Guidelines for hormone therapy in postmenopausal women. *Menopause*, 19(3), 257-271. https://doi.org/10.1097/gme.0b013e31824bdb2d

Zhu, X., & Liu, Y. (2018). Probiotics as therapeutic agents: A potential role in small intestinal bacterial overgrowth. *Gastroenterology Research and Practice*, 2018, Article ID 5024730. https://doi.org/10.1155/2018/5024730

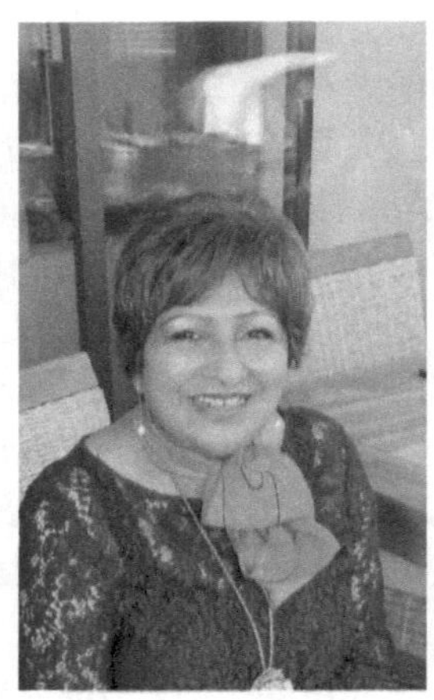

About the Author

Kareema Baksh – Managing Partner, Karah Capital Investments LLC

Kareema Baksh, with years of diverse experience, leads Karah Capital in multi-family real estate investments. Her background spans healthcare, franchise ownership, and functional nutrition, adding depth to her strategic planning and operational expertise. As a licensed insurance agent, she strengthens investment strategies with financial acumen. Actively involved in real estate groups, Kareema stays current with industry trends. At Karah Capital, she focuses on building sustainable wealth and community enrichment, viewing every investment as a partnership for mutual growth.

You can connect with me on:

🌐 https://karahinvestments.com
f https://www.facebook.com/kbakshali